Alternative Medicine Today

An A-to-Z Collection of 55 Natural and Holistic Treatments That Work

Ron Kness

Sneak Peek

One issue I have with modern medicine is that they tend to treat symptoms instead of getting to the root of the issue causing the symptoms. Many times, their solution is prescribing another pill. In many cases, there is a better way ... and that is the topic of this book: natural alternative ways that work independently or in conjunction with modern medicine that don't have the undesirable side effects. With some medications and treatments, the side effects are worse than the condition they are treating.

Specifically, in my book we look at three different types of natural treatments:

1. Alternative
2. Complementary
3. Integrative

We explain the difference between the three types, explain the nine benefits to using these natural therapies and introduce 55 alternative treatments and which treatment works best to treat a specific condition. Some of these alternative treatments are preventative in nature, meaning they are holistic on nature, so they are meant to keep you well, while others are aimed to get you well. The types of treatments range from A (acupressure) to Z (Zang-Fu) and everything in between.

If you are looking for ways to rely less on modern medicine and get back to using therapies and treatments that go back over 5,000 years and are still being used today ... because they work ... then this is a book you should have.

If you find an alternative treatment in it which looks promising for you, try it to see if it works. If unsure, consult with your doctor and see what s/he thinks. Some doctors are becoming more receptive to alternative-type, holistic treatments instead of prescribing another pill.

Table of Contents

Published by:

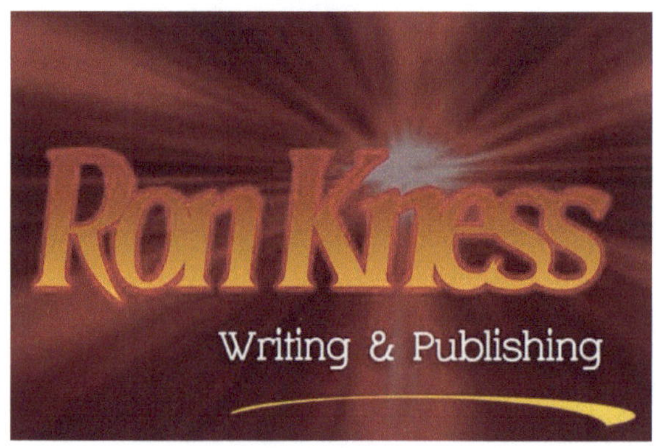

https://ronknesswriting.com

Ron Kness

San Tan Valley, AZ

United States of America

ISBN: 9781695620544

Disclaimer

This publication is for informational purposes only and is not intended as medical advice. Medical advice should always be obtained from a qualified medical professional for any health conditions or symptoms associated with them.

Every possible effort has been made in preparing and researching this material. We make no warranties with respect to the accuracy, applicability of its contents or any omissions.

See your healthcare professional before starting any diet, health or exercise program!

Introduction

According to Cancer.gov, *"complementary and alternative medicine (CAM) is the term for medical products and practices that are not part of standard medical care."*

Standard medical care is typically anything that is seen as conventional or traditional medicine as provided by health professionals with a license to practice medicine (M.D. or medical doctor or D.O. (doctor of osteopathy).

There are standard medicine practitioners who also practice CAM, as well as holistic practitioners who are medical doctors (M.D.) who treat patients within the principles set forth by holistic medicine.

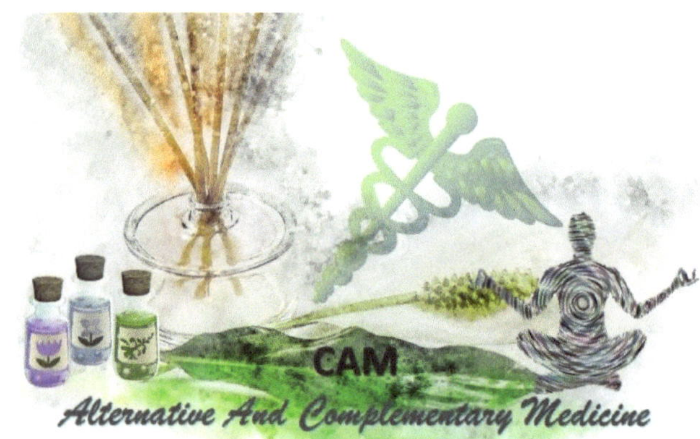

Alternative medicine can be a bit confusing. There are many categories, lots of techniques, and even lots of words in other languages associated with these methods of healing and promoting wellness. And what is alternative medicine an "alternative" to, anyway?

Understanding the basics of alternative medicine, as well as knowing about the various techniques and traditions that guide these methods, can help you determine how best to treat your health problems as well as remain healthy and strong.

This guide will dispel some myths about alternative medicine, provide you with a basic understanding of the most used alternative techniques, and help you understand all the benefits that you should consider when making health and wellness choices.

Let's start with a fundamental problem, which is understanding the difference between the many terms that get thrown around when talking about alternative therapies.

Alternative Versus Complementary Versus Integrative Medicine

There can be a lot of confusion when it comes to the many ways that alternative medicine techniques are categorized. Is it complementary? It is integrative? What does "alternative" actually mean? First, let's dispel all the confusion but looking at what these terms mean.

Alternative Medicine

The term "alternative medicine" is generally used to describe a treatment approach that replaces conventional medical care. It has become a catch-all term to mean anything that a typical medical doctor would not prescribe or advise, although this line is slowly becoming blurred as more and more alternative practices are becoming embraced by the mainstream medical establishment.

Complementary Medicine

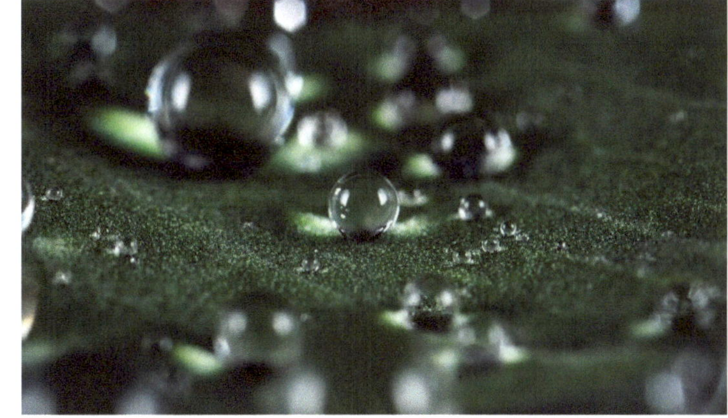

Complementary approaches to wellness are used in conjunction with, not instead of, more conventional methods of healing. Many of these techniques are identified as "alternative," but because they are used to complement the benefits of conventional medicine, they are labeled accordingly.

Here's an example to illustrate these terms. Fred is diagnosed with cancer. He decides to begin chemotherapy, which is a conventional medical treatment. He also uses music therapy to help him during his chemotherapy sessions and nutritional therapy to help his body get the nutrients it needs while it is battling the disease.

For Fred, the music and nutritional therapies are complementary to his conventional treatment.

Mike also has cancer and is choosing to treat his disease solely with acupuncture and homeopathy. For Mike, these two are alternatives to conventional medicine and therefore are alternative medical techniques. The same techniques could be considered either, depending on how they are used and if used in conjunction with conventional medical treatments or not.

Integrative Medicine

The National Center For Complementary And Integrative Health reports that this approach to healing combines both conventional and alternative choices together in a much more coordinated and thoughtful way, with a focus on holistically healing the patient.

Integrative medicine seeks to address the whole person, including the spiritual, emotional, and mental health as well as the physical well-being.

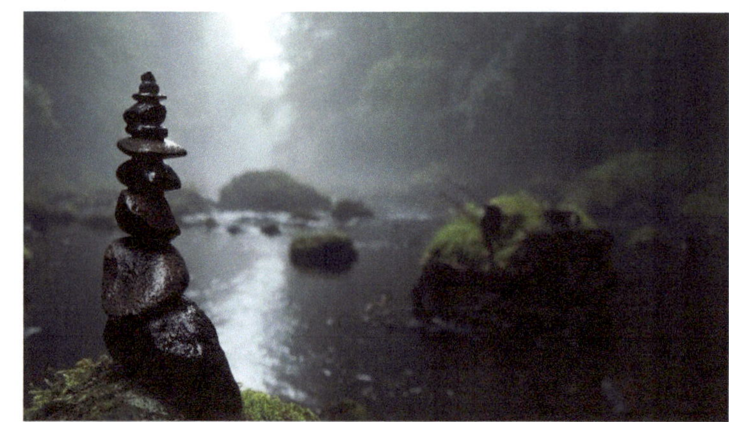

Treating the entire person involves multiple approaches and techniques, including those from both conventional and alternative medicine.

Building on our example from above, Steve also has cancer. Together, his oncologist, nutritionist, and hypnotherapist are coordinating a treatment plan that addresses Steve's many needs while he treats his illness. This is an integrative approach to wellness.

The Prevalence of Alternative Medicine in Use

Many people today claim to use some form of alternative or complementary therapy to manage their health. According to The National Health Interview Survey (NHIS), *"In the United States, approximately 38 percent of adults (about 4 in 10) and approximately 12 percent of children (about 1 in 9) are using some form of CAM."*

According to Grandview Research, 70% of adults surveyed in 2017 in the United States believe complementary and alternative medicine (CAM) provides positive results. 78% of those responders were women, and 62% were men.

In recent years, doctors and researchers have begun to include complementary and integrative approaches to medicine in their research to understand how alternative medicine is being used today.

According to the National Center For Complementary and Integrative Health,

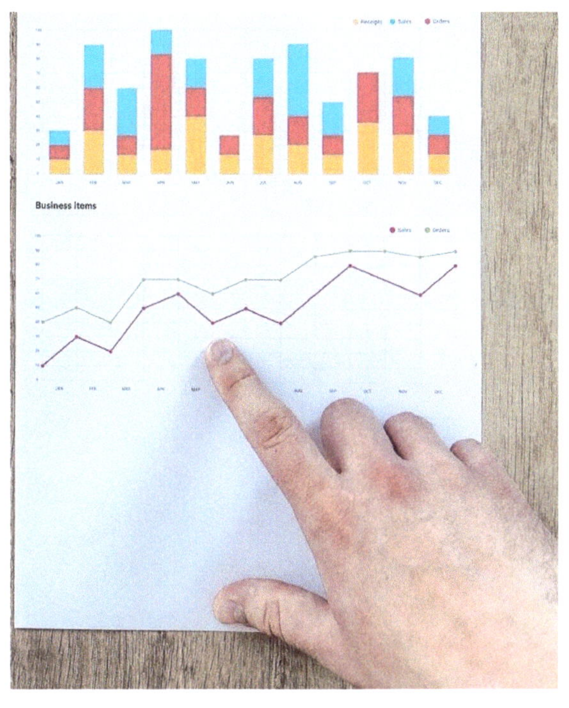

(https://nccih.nih.gov/research/statistics/2007/camsurvey_fs1.htm), Of those who use complementary or alternative medicine techniques, women are slightly more likely than men to use these techniques, and as income and education levels rise, so do the uses of these techniques. At least 40% of people in their 40s, 50s, and 60s are using some form of complementary or alternative approach for their health or wellness.

Use of complementary and alternative medicine is greatest among those of American Indian or Alaska Natives decent (50.3%), followed by whites (43.1%) and Asians (39.9%). Blacks and Hispanics are less likely to use these approaches (25.5 and 23.7% respectively).

When asked which complementary or alternative therapies they used, the most common responses included nonvitamin/nonmineral natural products, deep breathing, and meditation.

Among the top listed were also chiropractic care, massage, yoga, diet-based therapies, progressive relaxation, guided imagery, and homeopathy.

Many people report using natural products, which includes nutritional supplements and herbal remedies. The most popular of these in 2007 was fish oil supplements, and others high on the list include flaxseed, ginseng, and garlic.

People choose complementary or alternative medicine to address several health issues. Musculoskeletal problems, including back, neck, joint pain, and arthritis, are generally high on this list. Rounding out this list for uses of alternative medicines includes anxiety, high cholesterol, congestion, headache, and insomnia.

What Is Holistic Medicine

Now that we have a handle on these terms, let's examine a fourth that often appears when discussing alternative medicine. Where does holistic medicine fit in with all this? Holistic healing is not in place of alternative or complementary approaches.

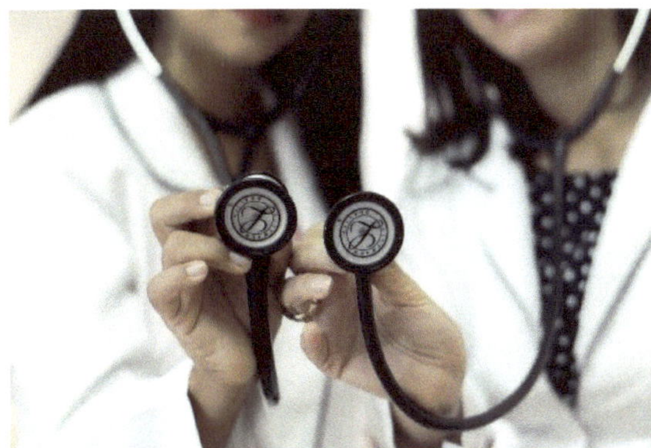

In fact, it could be a form of integrative medicine, as holistic healers seek to treat the whole person. In general, integrative approaches are used to treat a person when they are ill, while holistic approaches are used to keep you (or make you) healthy.

The goal of holistic medicine is your own optimal health and wellness. This is achieved by gaining proper balance in life, and treatment is based on addressing the interconnectedness between the various aspects of your life.

As a philosophy of wellness, holistic medicine is based on these ideas:

- Each person has innate abilities to heal themselves.
- The practitioner is treating a person, not a disease.
- Healing comes from a group effort of patient and doctor addressing many aspects of life that can change health outcomes.
- Any treatment should address the cause, not just symptoms.

A holistic doctor may use many different techniques and approaches to healing, from conventional to complementary to alternative, to help a patient achieve wellness. It's an integrative approach to wellness rather than disease management.

One of the greatest accolades of holistic medicine is that it can help prevent illness and chronic disease, as it often includes patient education on lifestyle and diet, self-care promotion, and use of medications in conjunction with complementary therapies.

9 Key Benefits Of Using Alternative Therapies

Grandview Research reports that *"the global complementary and alternative medicine market size was valued at USD 52.00 billion in 2017."*

Alternative therapies are used because they represent a different approach to healing, one that often focuses on balance, holistic healing, and restoring the body's natural energy. The most significant benefit of this form of healing is that is attempts to allow the body to heal itself while introducing therapies that will enable this to happen.

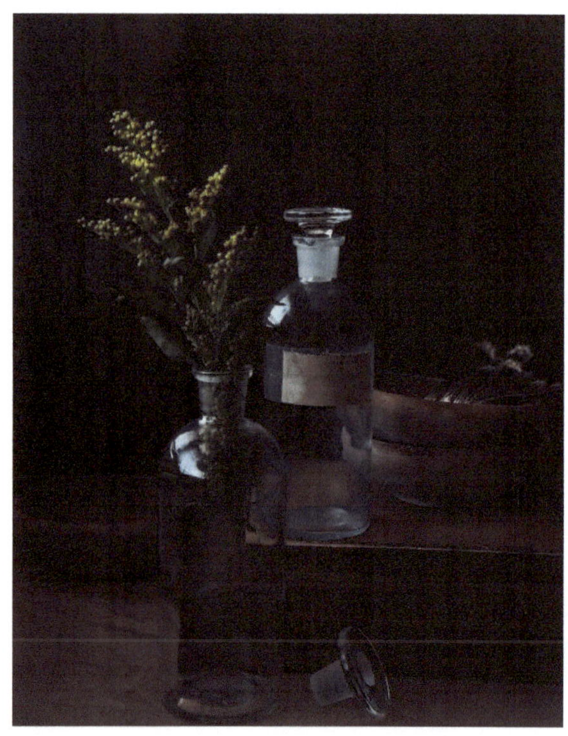

Most who seek alternative treatments do so to treat the whole body and to address root causes rather than merely mask symptoms.

Most people today see many different doctors who specialize in specific systems or diseases, and many long for an approach to health and healing that treats them as people with issues that may be interconnected. Most forms of alternative medicine focus on treating the whole person, not the illness.

Most alternative medical practitioners also spend more time with their clients or patients, which can be a welcome change from the typical 15-minute doctor's office visit these days. Some of them seem like they can't get you out of their office quick enough so they can get another patient in.

Personalized medicine means you can get a treatment plan based on your individual needs, and many people today appreciate the attention to wellness and overall health that alternative practitioners provide.

The significant benefit to alternative medicine is its focus on prevention.

While most conventional doctors only see you when there is a problem, your holistic medical professional will encourage you to come when you are well, too. What a novel idea! Prevention of disease is just as important as treatment, and alternative practitioners know this.

The key to selecting the right alternative or complementary therapy for you, or for looking for an integrative approach to healing, is to consider balance, your own priorities, and what you believe to be best for you.

Availability

One reason that many people use alternative medicine is that it is widely available. For example,

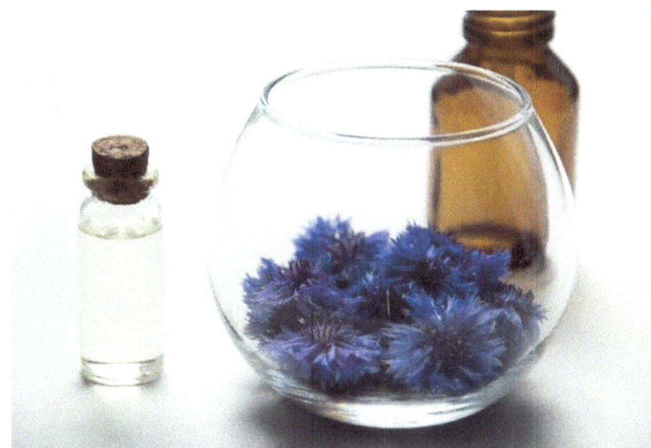

the use of herbs to maintain optimal health or to make home remedies, making it for more accessible and affordable for a wide range of people.

Mind body practices such as yoga and meditation can be easily practiced at home without the high costs often seen with

traditional medicine practices. My wife and I participate in a Hatha Yoga class once a week and it has helped with our flexibility and balance along with being more calming to the mind.

Affordability

A related reason is that alternative medicine is usually more affordable than conventional medicine. People who may have trouble paying for medical bills may be drawn to the comparatively low cost of alternative medicine. Our 1-hour yoga class costs us USD $5.00 each.

The cost of going to alternative medicine practitioners for services like acupuncture may be high but the cost of obtaining herbal supplements, essential oils, and other accoutrements of alternative medicine can be far more affordable than a trip to the hospital.

Natural Strategies in Healing

Prescription drug use is at an all-time high in the United States, and often patients complain that the first go-to of their doctor is to write a prescription.

Most all the therapies used in CAM are natural, this is far from the often chemically based interventions seen in conventional medicine. This includes, but is not limited to herbs, essential oils, diet, supplements, chiropractic treatment, mind-body practices and naturopathy.

This does **not** mean that CAM is a cure for any and all conditions, but it can offer a natural alternative and sometimes be a replacement of conventional medicine tools.

Improved Life Quality and Side Effects of Treatment

Another important reason people use alternative medicine is that it can improve life quality and lessen side effects of treatment. With some medications, the side effects are worse than the condition they are trying to treat.

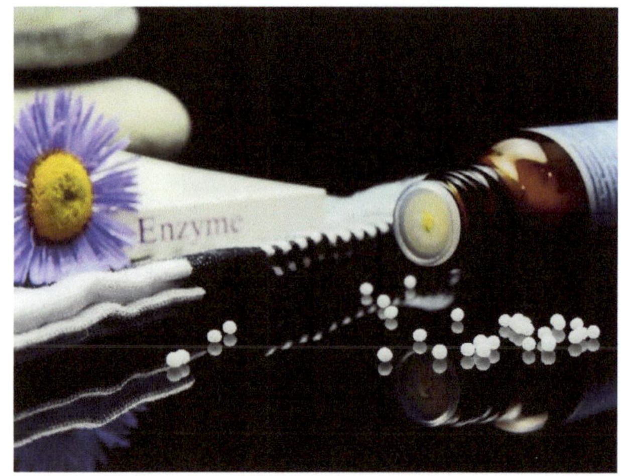

When people endure serious illnesses or chronic conditions, inevitably their life quality suffers, and side effects of conventional medicine treatments bring undue hardship. This is where CAM can help.

For example, Music Therapy is often used in pain management, which can be helpful for conditions such as arthritis and other chronic pain syndromes. Cancer.gov reports that acupuncture is helpful in reducing the side effects of treatment.

Trust

Millions of people all around the world genuinely trust alternative medicine as they have for the whole history of humanity. Some of the therapies used in CAM, including acupuncture, Ayurveda, homeopathy and herbalism have been in use for thousands of years, dating back to ancient civilizations. Eastern culture strongly believes in their effectiveness in the modern world.

A more accurate term for "alternative medicine" might be "folk medicine." "Folk" is usually used colloquially but it comes from the German word for "people," so "folk medicine" means something like "the people's medicine" or even "popular medicine."

Another reason that might shock skeptics of alternative medicine is that some proponents of alternative medicine are skeptical of institutionalized medicine. What this really comes down to is whether we should trust man-made and manufactured solutions more than we should trust natural solutions.

Many people lean toward alternative approaches because they are less invasive and produce fewer adverse side effects from most conventional treatments.

Modern medicine relies heavily on prescription drugs, whose list of possible side effects is often longer than its benefits. And modern medicine also tends to treat symptoms instead of getting to the source causing the issue.

55 Alternative Medicine Therapies A to Z

Acupressure

Acupressure was developed as a part of ancient Asian medicine, particularly Traditional Chinese Medicine. It has been used for over 5,000 years and involves the use of pressure from precise finger placements at different points on the body. The points that are used in acupressure are

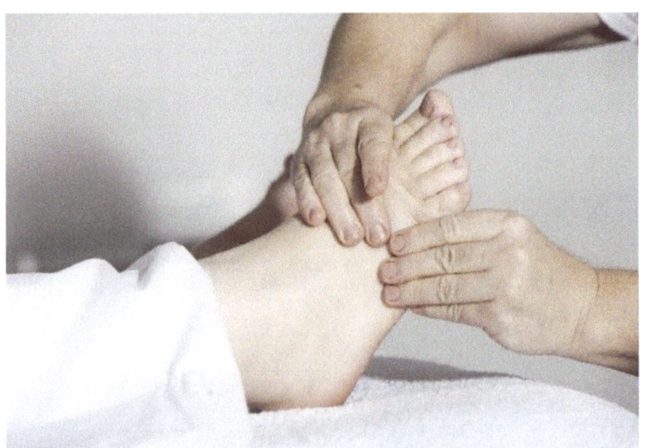

the same as those used in acupuncture and follow identified channels, which are called meridians. When activated by pressure, these points release life energy, which is known as "chi" ("qi" in Chinese).

Chi can release tension and improve blood flow. Using acupressure therapy is used to relieve pain, relax muscles, and enhance circulation. It can be applied to your own body or by a massage therapist or other practitioner of manipulative therapy. Acupressure can be used to help treat motion sickness, headaches, back pain, fibromyalgia, neck pain, and chronic fatigue. This form of alternative medicine is also used to treat many types of sexual dysfunctions and to enhance fertility.

Acupuncture

According to the Women's Health Research Institute at Northwestern University, *"At least 3 million adults nationwide use acupuncture every year."* Further, *"many well-designed studies have found that acupuncture can help with certain conditions, such as back pain, knee pain, headaches and osteoarthritis.*

Acupuncture, which was also introduced in Asia thousands of years ago, uses the same meridian channels as acupressure, but instead of using pressure, this technique releases chi using very fine needles.

Acupuncture is used in Traditional Chinese Medicine to treat, prevent, and even diagnose health problems. The needles, when placed in precise locations on the body, release your natural energy, which can help improve various ailments and conditions.

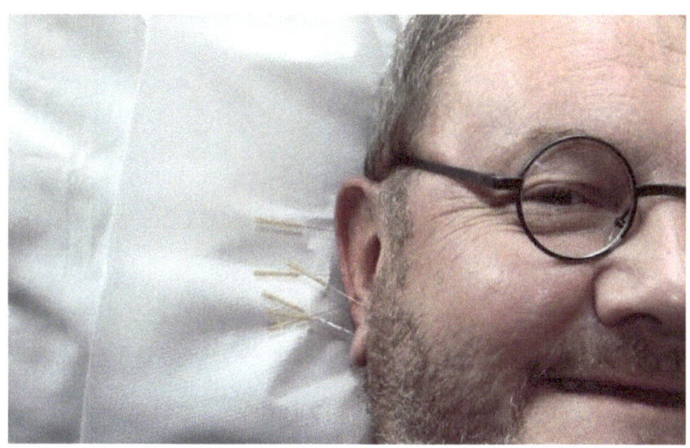

The goal of acupuncture is to restore the balance of your chi or energy flowing through your body. The benefits of this release of energy include all types of pain relief and treatment of many physical and emotional disorders.

According to Stephen Janz, author of the Evidence Based Acupuncture Evidence Project, *"It is no longer possible to say that the effectiveness of acupuncture can be attributed to the placebo effect or that it is useful only for musculoskeletal pain."*

According to Evidence Based Acupuncture website, *"The Acupuncture Evidence Project reviewed the effectiveness of acupuncture for 122 treatments over 14 clinical areas. They found some evidence of effect for 117 conditions. "Our study found evidence for the effectiveness of acupuncture for 117 conditions, with stronger evidence for acupuncture's effectiveness for some conditions than others. Acupuncture is considered safe in the hands of a well-trained practitioner and has been found to be cost-effective for some conditions. The quality and quantity of research into acupuncture's effectiveness is increasing"* (Acupuncture Evidence Project, p55).

The Evidence Based Acupuncture Project reports evidence of positive effects of acupuncture on the following conditions:

- Allergic rhinitis
- Chemotherapy induced nausea and vomiting
- Chronic lower back pain
- Headaches
- Migraine prevention
- Knee osteoarthritis
- Postoperative pain, nausea and vomiting

And evidence of 'potential positive effect' for more than 40 conditions including but not limited to:

- Anxiety
- Acute stroke
- Asthma in adults
- Cancer pain
- Depression
- Hypertension
- Obesity
- Sciatica
- Insomnia
- Irritable Bowel Syndrome
- Menopausal hot flashes
- Shoulder pain
- Smoking cessation
- PTSD
- And many more

It is important to look for a qualified and licensed acupuncturist who runs a clean office. Whenever possible get a recommendation from your physician.

Affirmative Prayer

Affirmative prayer is a method of positive worship that focuses on the desired outcome you wish to achieve. As a form of healing, affirmative prayer can help create the positive mindset necessary to achieve health and happiness.

Some refer to this as "spiritual mind treatment," as its purpose is to focus your thoughts to God so that they consistently and positively seek guidance for your improved health and wellness.

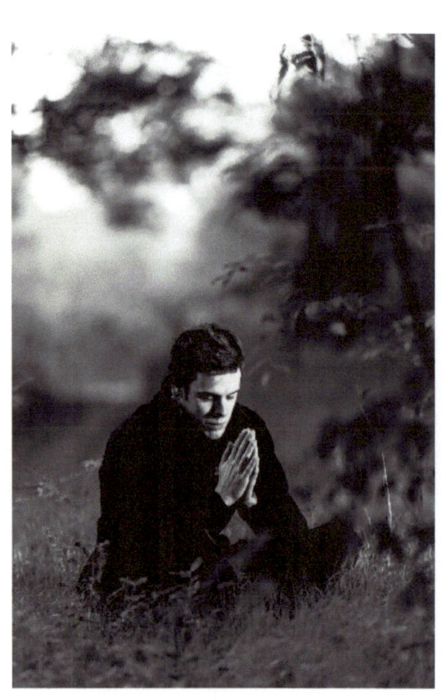

Affirmative prayer can be used by anyone seeking to connect spiritually with a higher power. Those with an illness can use this method of praying to focus intently on their desired state of health and their ideal outcome. Those with mental health struggles can also use affirmative prayer to gain strength and solace.

Alexander Technique

The Alexander Technique is a method whose purpose is to correct core posture that can cause many physical problems. The Technique educates its user about the importance of head, neck, and back alignment as well as proper posturing techniques.

Followers learn movement and poses that properly align muscles and unlearn poor habits of sitting, standing, and moving. Proper posture releases tension and remedies many medical issues.

Many who use the Alexander Technique are dancers, actors, and musicians, but anyone with chronic pain, muscle strain, headaches, or constant tension can receive help from this method.

When you learn to breathe differently and move your body for optimum posture, you will see improvement in your upper body in many ways. As you learn new habits and unlearn bad ones, you will practice breathing, walking, and engaging in everyday activities in new ways.

Applied Kinesiology

The study of body movements is called kinesiology, but applied kinesiology refers to muscle strength testing. This method is used to diagnose and treat medical problems based on the strength of various muscles.

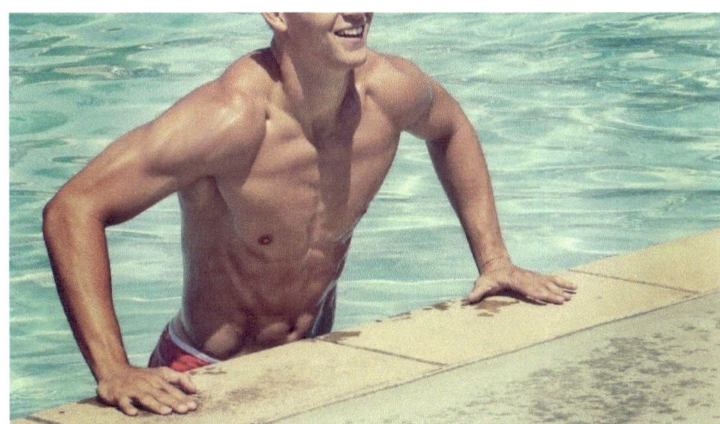

This branch of alternative medicine believes that various muscles within your body are linked to specific glands and organs.

When you have weakness in that muscle, this could be signaling problems, including hormonal imbalances, reduced blood flow, nerve damage, or other abnormalities. Applied kinesiology practitioners focus on correcting these muscle weaknesses to address the underlying issue.

Most use this technique to treat imbalances in the meridians used in traditional Asian medicines as well as address any problems of the nervous system or nutritional imbalances.

Many who practice this form of healing are chiropractors, but osteopathic doctors and others may also use it. Applied kinesiology has been used to treat headaches, diabetes, Parkinson's disease, and osteoporosis, just to name a few ailments.

Aromatherapy

Aromatherapy is the use of specific scents and fragrances to affect change in your physical or mental health. Most commonly, essential oils are used to supply scents that can influence mood and trigger physiological responses that can affect your well-being.

Essential oils contain the botanical essence of the trees, plants, and flowers from which they are distilled. The use of such scents to enhance mood and promote relaxation has been around for generations, but most recently, aromatherapy is being used to treat medical disorders.

Aromatherapy activates the brain's limbic system when your nose responds to specific scents. This limbic response leads to specific emotional and physiological changes, which can influence various organs, systems, and muscles.

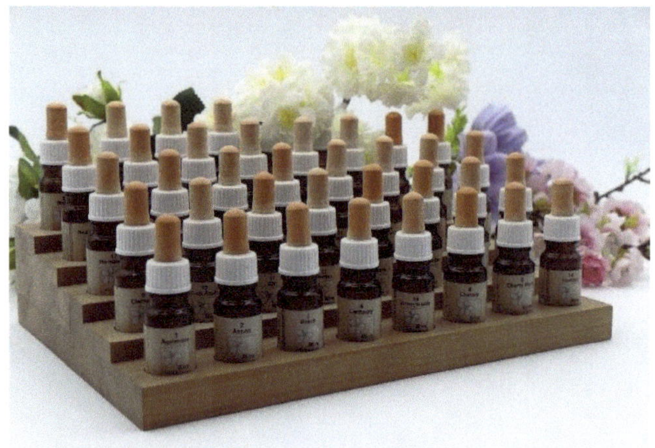

Medical aromatherapy can help address seizure disorders, diabetes, and other conditions. Most often, aromatherapy is combined with complementary treatments, including acupuncture and massage therapy.

Aromatherapy can be used to treat anxiety, sleep disorders, congestion, nausea, and even hair loss. Since the limbic system is so keenly activated with this form of treatment, it has a powerful effect on emotions, mood, and energy levels.

Autogenic Training

Autogenic training is a form of relaxation therapy that is used to reduce anxiety. It is especially helpful when addressing social anxiety disorder, which is also known as SAD. As a part of cognitive-behavioral therapy or used at home by the individual, autogenic training mimics the relaxed state many people experience while under hypnosis.

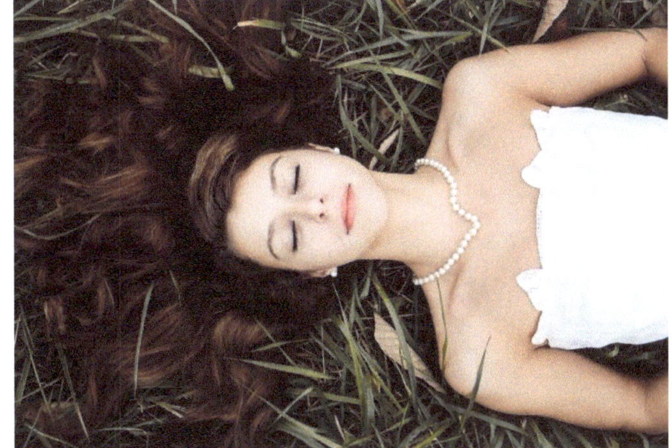

Users repeat various statements to themselves and engage in a process that brings warmth and heaviness to their bodies, which induces relaxation and reduces anxiety.

This form of relaxation is highly effective for treating anxiety, especially social anxiety. It can also reduce stress and promote calm, which can be helpful for those with sleeping disorders, mood issues, or other mental health challenges.

Ayurveda

Ayurvedic medicine, or Ayurveda, is among the oldest forms of holistic healing in the world, originating in India more than 3,000 years ago. Practitioners of Ayurveda believe there is a balance to be achieved between spirit, mind, and body to achieve wellness, and it looks to promote health rather than fight disease.

Ayurveda healers believe in the connection between a person and the earth as well as the interconnectedness of all the universe's elements- water, fire, air, space, and earth.

The goal of Ayurveda is to balance your doshas, or life forces, which are these elements in the human form. You have a Vata dosha, which combines space and air, a Pitta dosha, which combines fire and water, and a Kapha dosha, which combines water and earth. Every person's doshas are unique, with one being usually stronger than the others, and each dosha controls your essential body functions.

Ayurveda seeks to teach you to balance your doshas and to eat and live properly to maximize your health in order to live in harmony with the forces of the universe. Ayurvedic treatment is individualized to each person and its goal is to cleanse the body and restore harmony and balance. Practitioners will use techniques including massage, medicinal herbs, blood purification, enemas, and laxatives.

Biofeedback

One study (Biofeedback in medicine: who, when, why and how?; Frank, et al) is quoted as, *"Biofeedback therapy is a process of training as opposed to a treatment. Much like being taught how to tie their shoes or ride a bicycle, individuals undergoing biofeedback training must take an active role and practice in order to develop the skill. Rather than passively receiving a treatment, the patient is an active learner. It's like learning a new language."*

Biofeedback is a technique that strengthens the mind-body connection and uses an electronic cue to signal the need for a specific physiological response. This technique is used to influence your autonomic nervous system and create positive responses in heart rate, blood pressure, muscle tension, and other processes.

The electronic cues include beeps, visual images, and tones to signal special functions being measured, and you can use this information to check your health and facilitate the treatment of many different health issues.

According to Mayo Clinic biofeedback is used to manage the following:

- Anxiety
- Asthma

- Attention-deficit hyperactivity disorder
- Chemotherapy side effects
- Chronic pain
- Constipation
- Fecal incontinence
- Fibromyalgia
- Headache
- High blood pressure
- Irritable bowel syndrome
- Raynaud's disease
- Ringing in the ears (tinnitus)
- Stress
- Stroke
- Temporomandibular joint disorder
- Urinary incontinence

WebMD further explains why biofeedback appeals to many people:

- It is a noninvasive procedure
- It may reduce the need for and/or enhance the benefits of medication
- It allows people to feel more in control of their health

Biofeedback In Mental Health

Biofeedback is being aggressively researched and according to *Psychology Today* is a useful tool for psychologists in the mental health arsenal.

Psychology Today also quotes Carol Austad's (PhD psychologist at Central Connecticut State University) opinion of biofeedback, *"As an adjunctive aid to psychotherapy, it's fantastic,"* she adds. *"The patient feels as though they have control over their own bodily functions. When they have that feeling of mastery, you can accomplish more in psychotherapy." "Mind-body medicine is so prominent right now, and this is a way to help people learn mindfulness more quickly."*

Bio-Resonance Therapy

Bio-resonance therapy is a form of energy medicine that detects electromagnetic oscillations emitted by damaged or diseased tissues, then uses inverse frequencies to negate the effects of these cells.

Bio-resonance therapy begins with testing which uses 40 acupuncture points to measure the frequencies at various places in your body. This information is analyzed and interpreted to determine the source of your problem.

The principles that guide bio-resonance therapy rely on knowledge that all cells resonate at specific frequencies and that cells communicate using electromagnetic energy. When cells can communicate effectively with one another, you are more likely to remain healthy and strong.

Different resonant frequencies are detected for healthy versus unhealthy cells of the same tissue. When exposed to specific inverse frequencies, unhealthy cells will release wastes and toxins, which can lead to better health.

Bio-resonance therapy can be used to treat skin disorders, allergies, asthma, arthritis, and other inflammatory diseases. This therapy can help regulate hormones, detoxify the body, and improve overall cellular function.

Chiropractic Medicine

Chiropractic medicine involves the hands-on manipulation of the musculoskeletal structure, as well as other alternative treatments, to properly align the body and treat pain and other problems.

Chiropractic care is an example of an alternative medical treatment that has become nearly mainstream. Its techniques focus on the manipulation of the joints, bones, muscles, and connective tissues to restore alignment of the body.

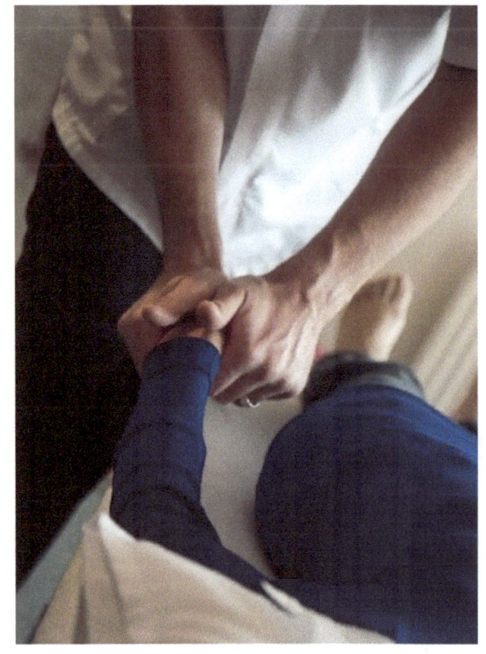

The most common and important benefit of chiropractic medicine is pain relief from injury, repetitive movement, or trauma. Chiropractic care can also be used to treat headaches, neck pain, fibromyalgia, and osteoarthritis.

Chromotherapy (Color Therapy)

Chromotherapy exposes specific points on your body to assorted colors of light in order to release your natural energy and evoke certain physical or emotional functions. All cells have

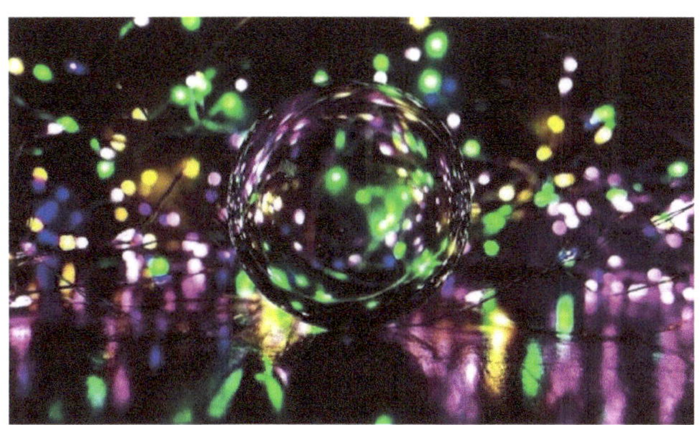

energy, and chromotherapy uses light energy to influence your spirit, consciousness, and soul in order to heal you and give strength.

Our bodies are consistently exposed to natural light, which is comprised of all colors, but sometimes, we need more of one color to help balance out what is happening inside our bodies and minds. Exposing yourself to different colors of light can help you regain balance and achieve better health.

Each color is used to benefit specific conditions or needs. For example, red can supply energy, so it is good for treating colds and fatigue. Yellow light stimulates happiness and helps spur digestion. Green calms, which is good for reducing inflammation as well as relaxing mood. Blue is a cool calm, which lowers blood pressure and can help you sleep better.

The use of colored light has been around for centuries, as people recognized the influence various colors have on your emotions and outlook. Practitioners use many different techniques to expose the eyes and skin to various shades to produce the desired effect.

Creative Visualization

Creative visualization is the use of the mind to bring about positive change in one's life. The technique involves using your imagination to think about your desired outcome, create its vivid existence in your consciousness, and attract your desired reality to yourself.

By thinking about what you want in life, you are more likely to be able to achieve it. And creative visualization influences even your subconscious mind, allowing you to alter your mindset and reality.

By harnessing the creative power of your thoughts, you first relax your body and empty your mind, then imagine your intended outcome. You should create a mental image of your ideal present, bringing those pictures to life with as much detail as possible.

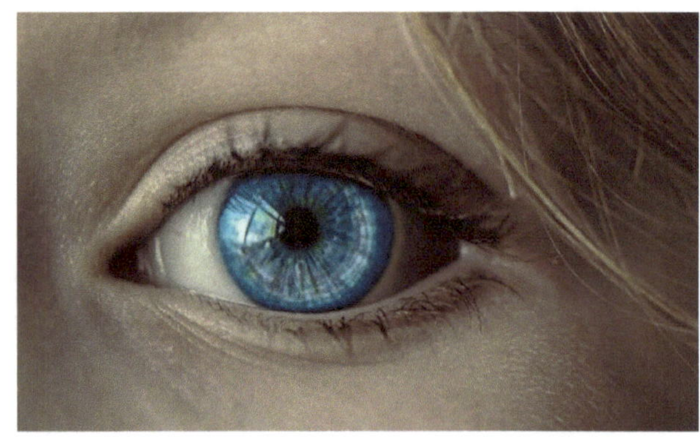

Then you feel the emotions you associate with this successful achievement. Your emotions bring this visualization into even clearer focus. Then, you believe that you have already achieved this outcome, that your visualization in indeed your present reality.

Creative visualization can help you carry out many health goals, including your mental and emotional well-being, overcoming fears, handling depression or anxiety, and learning to live with certain chronic illnesses.

Crystal Healing

Crystal healing uses the energy of specific stones or crystals to cure and protect against disease. Practitioners believe that gems and crystals can act as conduits to healing energy that can provide relief for some disorders.

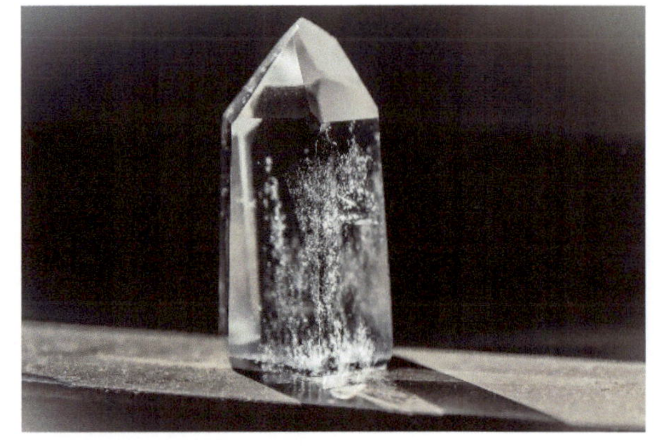

Most modern practices of crystal healing draw heavily from traditional Asian medicine techniques, including the understanding of chakras and chi, which connect the physical body to the natural and supernatural elements.

Each type of stone has specific qualities, and carefully chosen crystals are placed on specific points on the body, depending on your symptom or need. Treatment may always also involve wearing specific crystals on the body at all times, to protect against certain diseases or even negative energy. Some stones are believed to absorb positive energy, as well, and are often called talismans.

Cupping

Cupping is a technique that is used in Traditional Chinese Medicine. Special cups are filled with heated air, then placed on painful areas of the body. As the air inside cools and shrinks, a suction

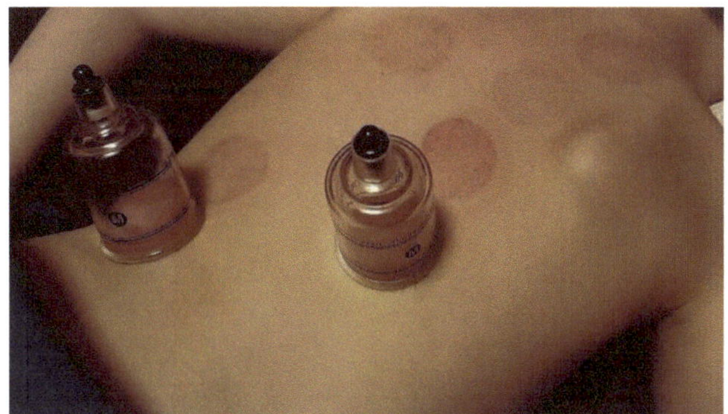

is created under the cup, increasing blood flow to this area.

This increased circulation can help with inflammation, pain, and other problems. Cupping is usually done by a trained acupuncturist.

This technique has been used for at least 2,500 years to treat respiratory ailments, pains, and aches. It also can relieve coughing, treat menstrual symptoms, and improve circulation. Once the cups are removed, a bruise often remains, and sessions are repeated once these marks disappear.

Ear Candling

Ear candling utilizes a hollow tube inserted into the ear, then heated. The tube, called the candle, is made from fibers, usually hemp or cotton. It is sometimes coated with beeswax. When a flame is applied to the end of the tub, the heat that is produced soothes and massages the ear, loosens compacted ear wax, and supplies relaxation.

Some people experience relief from earaches, sinus trouble, and headaches from this therapy. It is a very relaxing technique, so it can bring relief from tension or stress, as well. Candling does not remove excess ear wax but can loosen it so your body's natural processes can expel it.

EFT (Tapping)

EFT, which stands for Emotional Freedom Technique involves tapping on acupuncture points on your body as a treatment for specific phobias and fears. It is related to Thought Field Therapy, which proposes that negative emotions are the result of blocking energy from flowing through the body, and the tapping procedure acts as a trigger to unblock the flow of energy. This technique is also known as tapping.

Users are taught to tap specific points on their body, usually corresponding to points along meridians, that will release energy and block negative thoughts. Those who practice this report the end of their identified phobia. While treating fears is its most common use, some report that tapping can be used to treat all types of mental and emotional disorders.

Energy Medicine

 Energy medicine refers to many types of alternative healing practices that focus on activating or harnessing the energy of the body and the universe. Most energy medicine practices are meant to complement other treatments, whether alternative or traditional. The practices included under this broad umbrella term are used to facilitate healing through stimulation of the positive energy within.

Some examples of energy medicine, which you can learn more about within this book include therapeutic touch, Pranic healing, Reiki, and acupuncture. Each of these is used to treat different disorders or help with specific needs. Please read more about each therapy to understand its benefits.

Essential Oils

Essential oils are extracted from plants and contain the natural compounds, scents, and essences

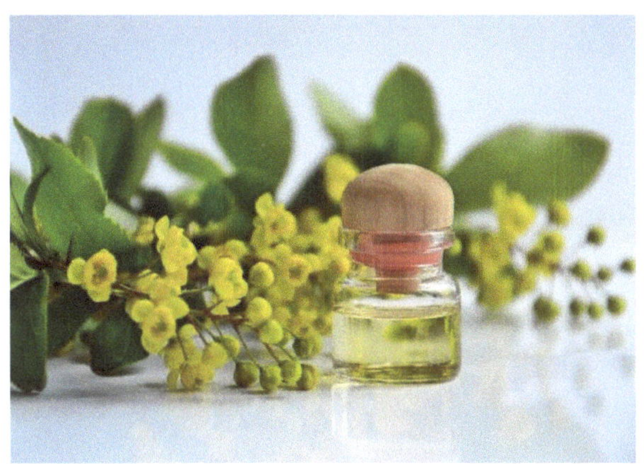

of the living plant. The unique properties of each essential oil come from which plant as well as which part of the plant was used in the extraction process.

Essential oils are extracted using distillation or cold pressing, and they are then combined with some carrier oil to make it ready to use. Any essential oil that is created using a chemical process will not have health benefits.

Essential oils are concentrated liquids that have the healing and curative properties of the plants from which they derive. Plants have been used for millennia to heal and prevent diseases.

 Oils can be used in lotions or creams to be applied topically, they can be used for aromatherapy, and some can even be ingested. Essential oils can alter mood, help with pain and inflammation, reduce anxiety or depression, and treat many different skin conditions. Some oils have antimicrobial compounds that can help treat infections, as well.

Faith Healing

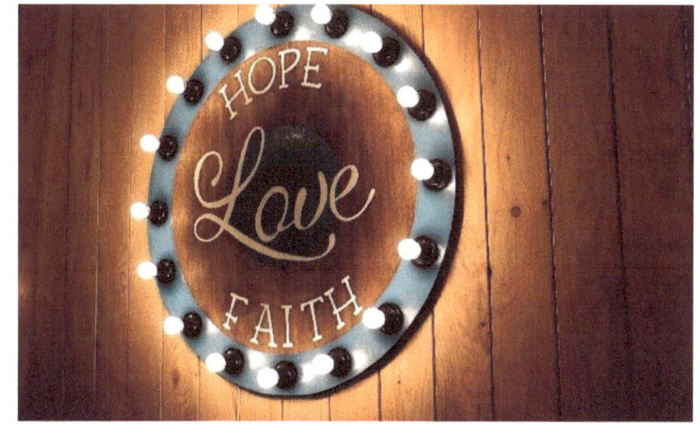

Faith healing, most simply, is the spiritual, mental, or physical healing of someone by the direct intervention of supernatural or divine power. The belief in prayer and the forces of divine intervention are said to be able to cure illness. This alternative practice involves healing touch, prayer, and other techniques to connect one with their religious or spiritual beliefs and provide relief from ailments or problems.

Faith healing can cure any illness, according to believers. It is used widely in many cultures to treat several diseases and disorders.

Herbalism

Also known as phytotherapy, herbalism is the use of plants to address ailments and to promote wellness. This type of medical practice has been around nearly as long as man, and almost four-fifths of the planet still rely on herbal remedies and medicine to treat some or all their diseases.

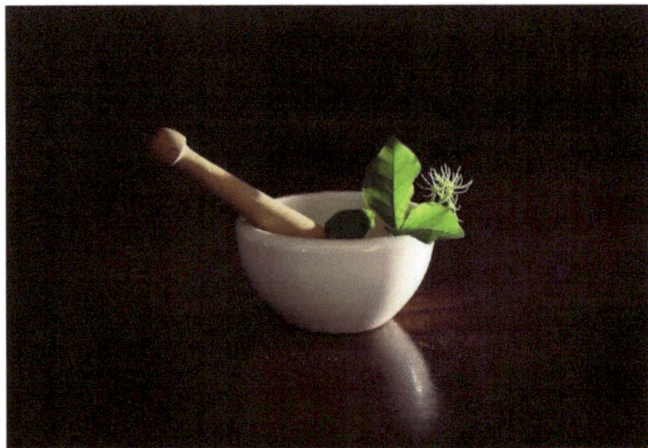

In fact, half of all prescription drugs contain ingredients derived directly from plants, and our current medical knowledge is based on a foundation of herbal medicine.

Herbalism utilizes the natural compounds found in plants to treat illnesses non-invasively and non-aggressively. Herbs, which can include the roots, stems, flowers, and other plant parts, allow your body's natural processes to work more efficiently, enabling you to heal yourself. Herbalism prefers to approach healing from a holistic standpoint and will focus on all aspects of wellness.

Herbalism can be used to treat any number of ailments, disorders, and conditions. A trained herbalist will tailor a specific treatment plan to your needs.

Homeopathy

Homeopathy, which is also called homeopathic medicine, is a system of alternative medicine that uses small doses of various medicines to treat a wide range of illnesses. Homeopathy is based on three important principles.

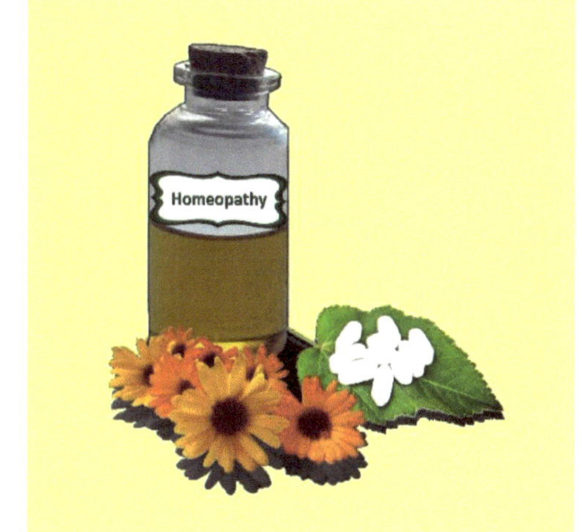

The first is the law of similars, which says that a cure will create symptoms similar to the ailment. The next is the principle of a single remedy, which means that one medicine should cover all the problems you are experiencing. The final is the principle of the minimum dose. This includes giving medicine in small doses, and dosage should start very small until it is clear the effect it has on the symptoms.

Homeopathic medicines are made from plant, animal, mineral, and synthetic substances, and they are diluted to create very weak concentrations. These homeopathic therapies are used to treat skin conditions, pain, digestive disorders, and other ailments. Some chronic but not serious conditions, like ear infections, can also receive help from homeopathy.

Hypnosis

Hypnosis, which is known as hypnotherapy or trance work, involves techniques to foster healing

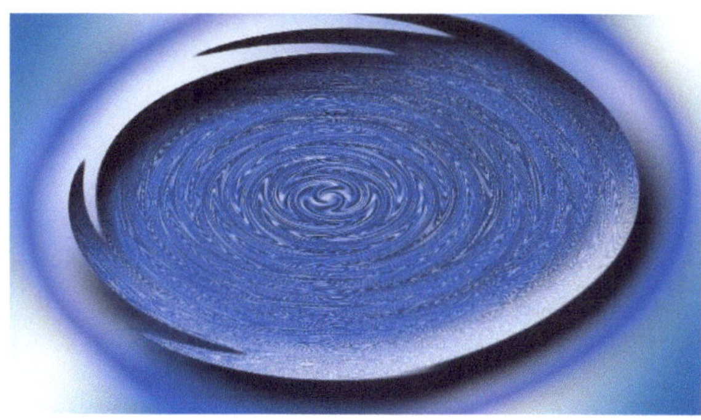

through a stronger body-mind connection. A trance, in which you are in an altered state of conscious, can increase your awareness and help you receive suggestions to alter your state and promote better health. You must choose to enter a hypnotic state, and while you can use a therapist to guide you, self-hypnosis is also possible.

During a trance, suggestions are offered which can help remove any psychological obstacles and strengthen your sense of self, which can help you change your behavior. Hypnosis can be used to treat a wide variety of ailments and problems.

Hypnosis can help with gastrointestinal disorders, skin problems, and any disorder that is caused by or made worse by stress. Other uses for hypnosis include weight loss, smoking cessation, and any other issue where willpower and motivation are needed for success. Hypnosis can help with sleeping disorders, autoimmune diseases, and anxiety.

Light Therapy

Known also as bright light therapy and phototherapy, light therapy uses full-spectrum lights to mimic sunlight to treat various disorders. Lightboxes that emit bright light can help those who live in areas with little sunlight or those who cannot get outside regularly.

Light therapy is mainly used to treat Seasonal Affective Disorder (SAD), which is a type of depression that results from reduced sun exposure during colder months with shorter days. Therapy involves sitting in front of a light box for up for 30 minutes each day, exposing skin and eyes to full-spectrum light.

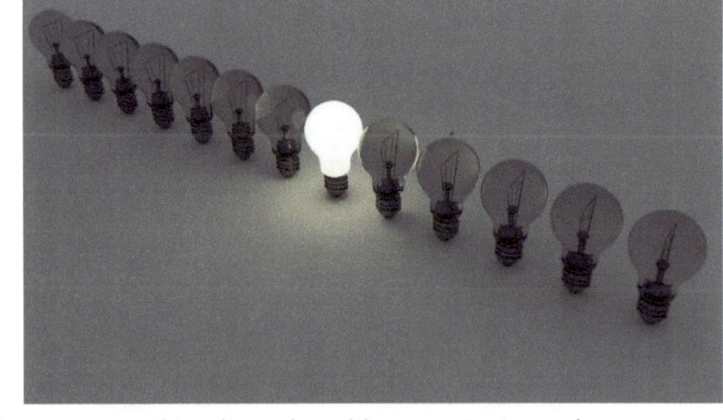

Light therapy affects the brain's chemicals that regulate mood, which makes it an effective treatment for this form of depression. Other types of light therapy use only ultraviolet (UV) wavelengths to treat skin disorders like psoriasis and some types of skin cancer.

Light therapy may be a safe alternative to antidepressants in some suffering from SAD. It has also shown to be helpful in treating insomnia, PMS, jet lag, and even obsessive-compulsive disorders.

Magnet Therapy

 Magnet therapy utilizes magnets placed on the body to treat disease and reduce pain. This form of alternative medicine includes magnetic field therapy as well as bioenergy therapy. Magnets of

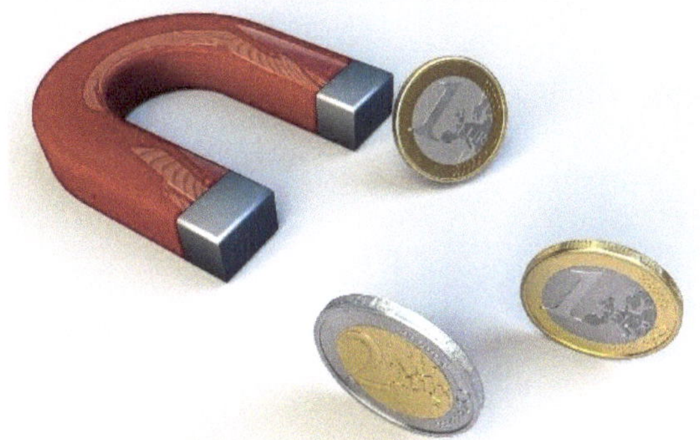

varying strengths are placed or worn on the body, used inside braces, or held to the body using adhesive patches, and the magnetic fields are said to stimulate cell activity. The influence of magnets on cells can improve circulation, enhance oxygen levels, and promote healing.

Conditions that are most often treated with magnet therapy include circulatory problems, inflammatory disorders, nerve disorders like diabetic neuropathy, insomnia, several types of pain, stress, and fibromyalgia.

Manipulative Therapy

 Manipulative Therapy, also known as Osteopathic Manipulative Treatment (OMT), involves a hands-on technique for diagnosis, treatment, and prevention of disease and injury. Manipulative therapy is usually performed by an osteopathic physician (DO) and involves moving joints and muscles on the body as well as stretching and applying pressure to the body.

The goal of OMT is to understand the connection between muscles, bones, and nerves and how these influence various systems and processes.

Manipulative therapy is safe for use with people of all ages, and it can reduce the need for certain medications or procedures in many cases. It is often used to treat carpal tunnel syndrome, migraines, menstrual pain, asthma, or to treat any number of alignment and structural issues with your musculoskeletal system.

Massage Therapy

Massage therapy is widely recognized as an excellent tool for relaxation, but the manipulation of your soft tissue is also beneficial to your health in other ways. Massage is a hands-on technique

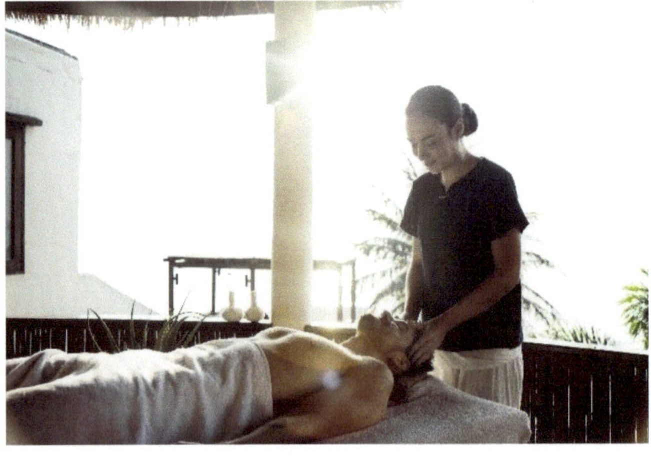

that involves the manual manipulation of your muscles, tendons, ligaments, and other connective tissues with a goal of enhancing your well-being and health.

There are many different methods and types of massage, each with a specific purpose or use. Massage not only releases tension in muscles but also can rehabilitate injured tissues, lower pain and inflammation, and reduce anxiety.

Massage therapy is used to promote relaxation, but it also can be used for the treatment of mental health disorders like depression and anxiety. It can help with certain skin conditions, pain disorders, dementia, and Parkinson's disease, too. It can even help enhance fertility and be used to promote the health of pre-term infants.

Meditative Movement

Meditative movement includes any type of meditation that involves moving. There are many different techniques that are classified as moving meditation, including Tai Chi, yoga, and Qi gong. If you apply mindfulness principles and the right pace, just about any movement can be made meditative, though.

This form of meditation is an excellent alternative for those who prefer a more active way to

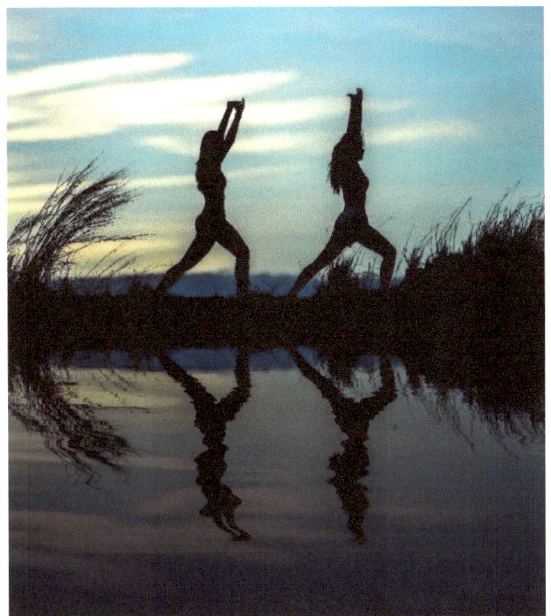

meditate. Meditative movement provides a release of tension and increased blood flow while also engaging in mindful thought.

In general, meditative movement involves paying attention to your actions as well as the flow of energy through your body.

You focus your attention on either a particular part of your body, such as your feet, or your body as a whole. Movements are kept slow to help with focus and attention, and you still are focused on your

action and its effect on your body throughout the practice.

The goal of meditative movement is to focus your mind and attention, to become more mindful, and to move beyond your own mind to experience your essential nature. Doing so can promote happiness and peace, reduce stress, help you become more aware of yourself, others, and your life, and enjoy your life more. Meditative movement also helps you stay connected to your body's needs, which can lead to improved health overall.

Meridians

As discussed previously, meridians are commonly used in Traditional Chinese Medicine (TCM), as well as other, ancient medicinal practices. They are specific channels or pathways within your body that move and release energy. Your chi, or vital life energy, flows through these meridians. Blocking your chi can cause illness or pain.

Acupressure and acupuncture, as well as other techniques, use points along these meridians. Pressure, needles, or other stimulation is applied to these points to rebalance and correct your flow of chi. Within TCM, there are over 300 points found on the various meridians in the body.

Practitioners of TCM have identified 12 regular meridians, each of which corresponding to an organ and run through the body to either a foot or hand.

The heart, lungs, spleen, liver, and kidneys are called yin organs and are linked to a yin meridian, while the intestines, stomach, bladder, and gallbladder are yang organs connected to a yang meridian.

The meridians carry energy in a specific path throughout your body and understanding your ailment will allow the activation of various points along these meridians to encourage energy flow, which links to your health and ability to heal.

Mind-body Practices

Mind body practices incorporate the use of the mind with movement to yield many different benefits for mind, body and spirit.

Meditation

Meditation is a practice that dates back thousands of years to ancient India. In modern, times millions of people meditate regularly and for many great reasons. Numerous scientific studies have found meditation to provide very real and verifiable benefits for mind, body, spirit and even anti-aging benefits for the brain.

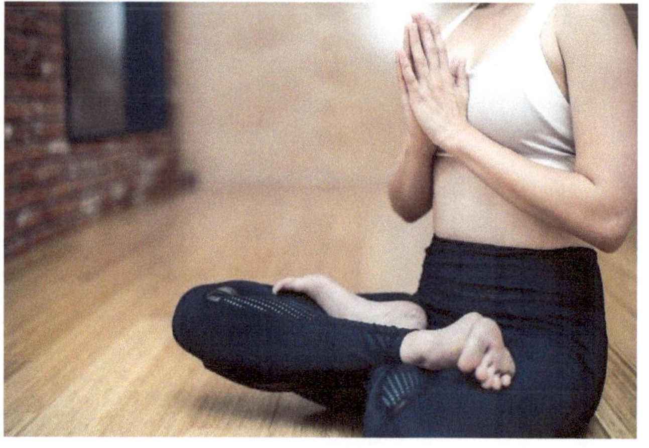

Some of the key benefits include

- Stress management
- Reduce anxiety
- Improved emotional health
- Higher levels of body awareness, so helps with diet control and self-care needs
- Greatly enhanced self-awareness
- Slows aging in the brain by increasing its white matter
- Boosts attention, focus and concentration

- May help prevent dementia and reduce age-related memory loss
- Calms the mind
- Better sleep
- Lower blood pressure
- Improved relationships due to a deeper connection to self and self needs
- Pain management

Tai Chi

Tai chi is a form of meditative movement. It originated in China, and while there are several unique styles of practice, they all have the same guiding principles. These include integrating the

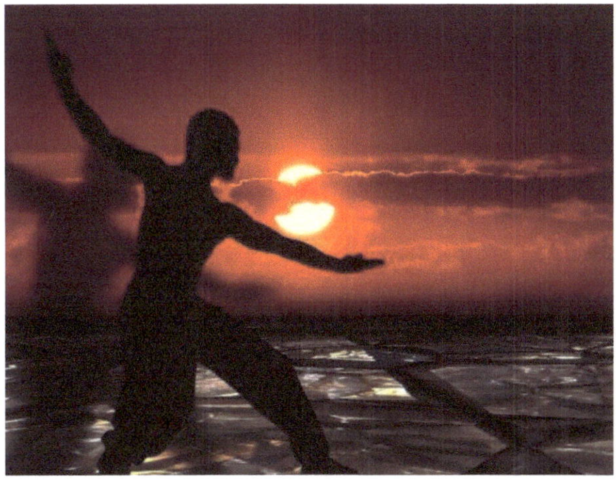

body with the mind, controlling your movements and breath, creating internal energy, being mindful, loosening your body, and seeking serenity.

The movements of tai chi are performed to cultivate your chi and allow it to flow smoothly and powerfully through yourself.

Tai chi builds muscle strength, boost your immunity, improves your flexibility, and relieves pain while reducing stress. The meditative movements teach you focus and attention, provide emotional tranquility, and connect you to your spirit.

Yoga

According to the National Center For Complimentary and Integrative Health, *"Yoga was the most commonly used complementary health approach among U.S. adults in 2012 (9.5%)."* Heart.gov reports that 21 million adults and more than 1.5 million children practice yoga.

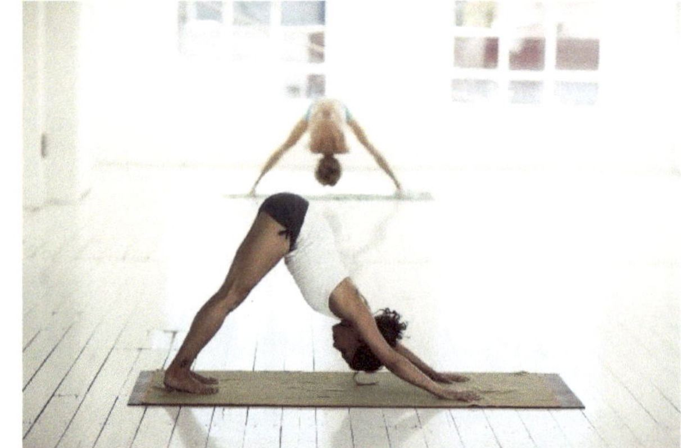

Yoga has come to mean many things in today's world, but it essentially a meditative movement that promotes a connection between the mind, body, and spirit.

The techniques of yoga were introduced in India over 5,000 years ago, and it is a system of philosophy and practice that is designed to promote peace of mind, mental clarity, and spiritual growth as well as physical wellness.

The techniques of yoga are meant to guide your life for better living. They take intense study to understand fully, so a simple weekly yoga practice is not enough to fully grasps its nuances.

However, using yoga techniques like Hatha yoga can help you relax, become more mindful, and connect with your health and wellness.

Yoga is not just something you do with your body; it is a way to greatly improve health and wellness on many levels. According to healthline.com, it can:

- Stress management
- Calms the mind and body
- Lowers blood pressure
- Lowers pulse rate making the heart work more efficiently
- Improves blood oxygenation)
- Pain management, including, chronic back pain, Fibromyalgia and arthritis

WebMD has this to say:

- Improves blood circulation, which improves cognitive function and memory
- Lung health
- Digestive health
- Reduces anxiety
- Stronger immunity
- Relaxation of mind and body
- Evidence finds yoga may lower blood glucose
- Stimulates the body's detoxification process that may delay aging
- Improved body awareness though the mind-body connection

Other health websites add to this by saying:

- Improves posture and flexibility (www.hopkinsmedicine.org)
- Good for muscle health (www.hopkinsmedicine.org)
- Heart health (everydayhealth.com)
- Builds strength (www.hopkinsmedicine.org)
- Better sleep (www.hopkinsmedicine.org)
- Improved balance and stability (www.hopkinsmedicine.org)
-
- Stronger core (www.hopkinsmedicine.org)
- Improved body control (www.hopkinsmedicine.org)
- Better life quality, improved mood for sufferers of chronic diseases, such as heart disease (heart.gov)
- Improved cardiovascular health (heart.gov)

Conditions/Diseases Helped By Yoga

WebMD confirms the following conditions to be helped by yoga

- Carpal tunnel syndrome

- Menopause symptoms

- Back pain

- Asthma

- Cancer treatment side-effects

- Migraines

- Obsessive compulsive disorder

Qi Gong

Qi gong, also known as qigong and chi kung, is a type of meditative movement aimed at improving your mental and physical health. It does this by integrating movement with posture, breathing, sound, focused intent, and self-massage.

There are many ways to practice qi gong, including many traditions and lineages. The purpose of the practice is to open the flow of energy in your meridians, enhancing your ability to feel and experience your life force as well as the forces of the universe. It is a series of slow, gentle movements that warms and tones tissues, promotes circulation, and helps you attend to your needs.

Qi gong is a meditative movement technique that can be used by anyone wishing to practice mindfulness, reduce stress, or become more connected to their body. The various paths of qi gong can be used for personal cultivation and to enhance well-being.

Music Therapy

According to the American Music Therapy Association, *"music therapy interventions can focus*

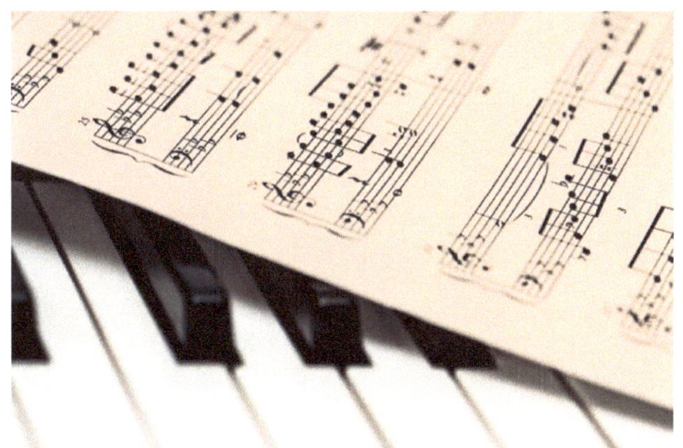

on pain management for physical rehabilitation, cardiac conditions, medical and surgical procedures, obstetrics, oncology treatment, and burn debridement."

Music therapy, when used in a clinical setting, is used to help patients reach their individual goals. By addressing physical, psychological, or cognitive challenges through music, the patient is able to clearly identify their behavior.

The American Music Therapy Association reports music therapy helpful in:

- Reducing stress and anxiety
- Alleviating pain
- Improved blood pressure
- Improved respiration
- Lower heart rate and boosts in cardiac output
- Relaxes muscle tension

Music therapy uses music to heal and provide care for individuals. In a therapy session, music is used in a variety of ways to reach someone emotionally, mentally, or physically. Music therapy can involve singing, listening, exercising, meditating, and even playing instruments by participants.

Music connects with many parts of your mind, including your emotional response center, and using music in therapy can help enhance mood, boost cognition, and aid in relaxation.

Music therapy is used in a wide variety of settings and with people of all ages and abilities. It can be used for emotional pain and stress, to treat stress-related disorders, to improve sleeping disorders, and to treat mental illness.

It has also been used successfully to help those with autism, learning disorders, eating disorders, communication disorders, and those with a history of abuse or trauma. It allows participants to express emotions without words, can give the participants confidence, promotes concentration, and can even help with memory issues.

If you're looking for a qualified music therapist, it's best to look for someone who is Board Certified in Music Therapy.

Naturopathy

Naturopathy is a system of treating someone using diet, exercise and other natural approaches and eschewing medications and prescription drugs. Naturopaths use natural therapies to allow

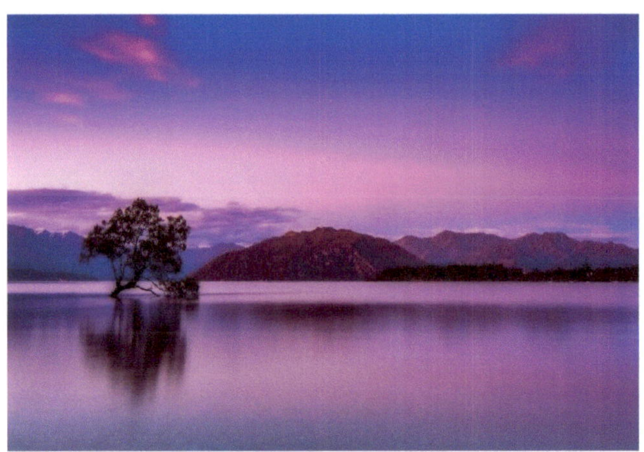

the body to heal itself. This form of alternative medicine treats the whole person and focuses on healing the cause of any illness, not just addressing symptoms.

A visit with a naturopath could take up to two hours, as the practitioner examines you, asks questions, and tries to understand your lifestyle.

Education and prevention are two main goals of naturopathic medicine, with a focus on nutrition, exercise, stress management, and lifestyle choices related to your overall health and well-being.

Naturopaths use many different treatment options, including herbal medicine, acupuncture, touch therapy, and other alternative approaches, to address problems in your health.

Naturopathy is used to treat all types of disorders and illness as well as promote overall health and well-being.

Neuro-Linguistic Programming (NLP)

Neuro-linguistic programming (NLP) is a technique that teaches you to learn and carry out new tasks by analyzing successful people and applying their techniques to your life. The principle behind this therapy is that, if you can understand how someone else accomplishes something, you can learn and copy their technique, giving you a chance to be successful, too.

The technique can be used to learn language, patterns of behavior, mindsets, or anything that can be experienced. The purpose of NLP is to learn a systematic approach to learning and experiencing life so that you can always be getting feedback and setting new goals for yourself.

This technique is popular as an approach to helping those in business, the performing arts, sports, and medicine, where you want to learn from the success of others and continue to refine your practice over time.

Therapists who use NLP methods try to understand the behavioral and thinking patterns of patients, then recommend new behaviors that would replace unproductive ones. NLP can help people with different mental health conditions, including depression, PTSD, panic disorders, phobias, and addiction.

Nutritional Healing

Nutritional healing is a therapy that uses supplements, herbs, and food to treat various disorders and ailments. By maximizing the nutritional powers of plants, vegetables, fruits, and other foods, you can help your body heal itself. In addition to eating certain foods, this form of

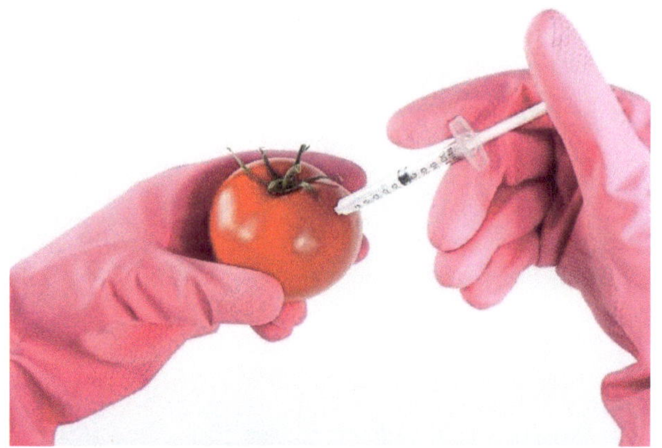

healing also uses fasting or abstinence from specific foods, as well as topical applications of certain foods, to address various issues.

Strategic eating and managing your diet are believed to reverse many physical ailments, including cardiovascular disease, inflammatory disorders, and respiratory diseases. Even symptoms of certain mental health conditions can be mitigated by the right nutrition.

Nutritional healing is also helpful for limiting symptoms from certain chronic diseases like Celiac disease and diabetes. Healthy nutrition can also help boost your immune system and allow you to fight off other conditions and diseases.

Nutritional Supplements

Nutritional supplements, also known as dietary supplements, are manufactured products that supplement various nutrients that may be missing from your diet.

Supplements can be in the form of powder, tablet, capsule, or liquid, and these are meant to provide you with essential nutrients that are otherwise missing or too low in the foods you normally consume.

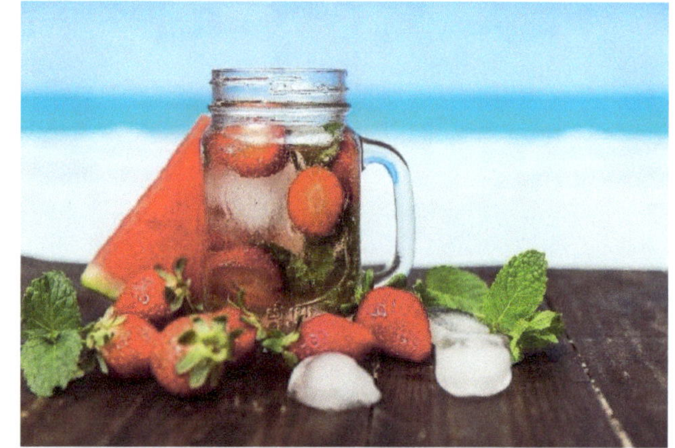

Supplements may provide you with amino acids, fatty acids, fiber, minerals, vitamins, or a combination of these.

Nutritional supplements are generally considered inferior to natural foods but preferred to nutritional deficiencies. Not only are they effective for those whose diets may lack specific compounds, but they are also necessary for people with certain diseases or disorders.

Pregnant women, the elderly, and those with a poor appetite due to medical problems may need supplements to get all they need for optimal health. If you have food allergies or follow a specific elimination diet, such as veganism, you may lack specific nutrients in your diet.

Osteopathic Medicine

Osteopathic medicine is a type of healing that is patient-focused and deals with all aspects of patient care, including spiritual, mental, and physical well-being. Practitioners focus on wellness and treat problems holistically. Osteopathic care addresses the relationship of organs and systems to muscles and bones as well as the mind.

This form of medicine is preferred by those who wish to focus on preventative care, holistic healing, and treating the cause of disorders, not just the symptoms. While osteopathic practitioners use some conventional medical techniques, they also rely on some more alternative choices, as well.

Polarity Therapy

Polarity therapy, based on the principles of attraction and union of opposites across a middle point, stimulates and balances the flow of energy within the body. Your body is an energy system, similar to a magnet.

You have positive and negative currents that flow through your body as well as poles that anchor your energy. Polarity therapy works to focus the flow of your chi, or life energy. The flow of this energy leads to better health and overall well-being.

Polarity Therapy is a combination of techniques, including counseling, nutrition, exercise, and bodywork to help you achieve optimal health. The emphasis on this form of therapy is on self-responsibility.

Pranic Healing

Pranic healing involves the cleansing of one's aura, which is the energy field that extends from your body. Life experiences and events can damage or congest this energy field, and this technique uses a no-touch method to release the flow of energy (prana) through your aura.

Pranic healing is generally used to complement other therapies, and it can serve to boost your body's own ability to heal itself. It is often used to treat chronic stress, boost mood, clear negative emotions, reduce pain, and improve your ability to heal yourself and promote personal wellness.

Psychic Surgery

Psychic surgery is the channeling of spirit surgeons to perform the removal of physical and emotional damage from the body. No incision is made by the psychic surgeon. Instead, the spirit surgeon enters the body to remove diseased tissue or heal emotional wounds.

Reflexology

Reflexology, sometimes called foot reflexology, applies pressure to specific points on the hands or feet to promote relaxation, improve circulation in the body, and restore function to various systems.

The technique is based on a belief that the nerves in your extremities are linked to specific areas of your body and placing pressure on these points can release energy and promote healing in those areas.

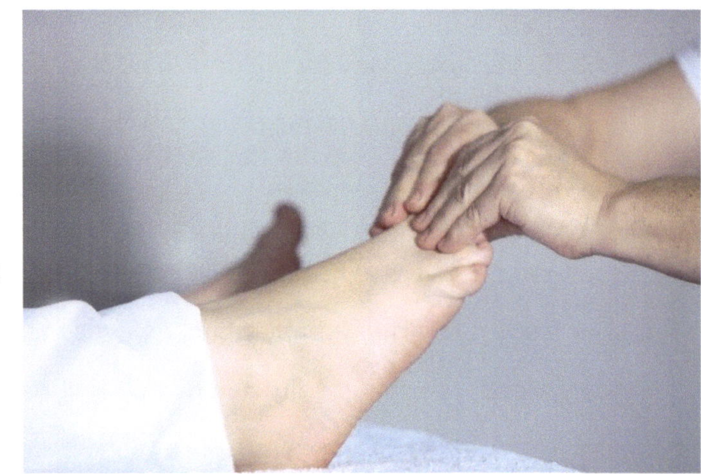

Pressure on the feet and hands is ultimately very relaxing. While relaxation is a genuine benefit of this technique, it can also be used to help treat neuropathy in the lower body, reduce stress, treat arthritis pain, reduce hypertension, and help with symptoms of depression and anxiety. Reflexology aims to improve circulation, which is also helpful for several pain and inflammatory disorders.

Reiki

Reiki, a technique that originated in Japan, translates to "spiritually guided life-force energy." The practice channels life force energy, or chi, (ki in Japanese), through the hands and onto someone else.

It is used to heal physical and mental trauma and provide spiritual support to another. Reiki practitioners are trained to place their hands over affected areas, causing the negative energy to release, taking away any physical, emotional, or psychological pain.

Reiki has many benefits, with the most important being relaxation, which can allow your body to focus on its own healing processes. When you can relax and focus, you can relieve stress, cope with your pain or problem, and improve your well-being.

Reiki has been used to treat pain, neurodegenerative disorders, fatigue, sleeping disorders, inflammatory diseases, and mental health issues like anxiety and depression.

Shiatsu

Shiatsu, the Japanese word for finger pressure, is a type of bodywork similar to acupressure. Shiatsu is often used to describe a type of massage, but it can be used in other applications. The finger pressure of shiatsu releases your chi (ki), disrupting disease and restoring health.

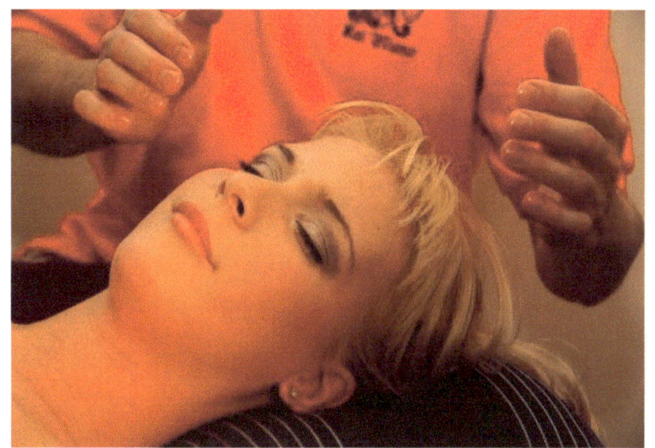

Shiatsu restores energy to specific areas by either stretching or pressing on various points along your meridians. This technique improves blood flow and releases cellular waste and toxins, which can help you heal and feel better.

Shiatsu not only lifts your mood, but it can also be used to help you relax, deal with emotional or mental health issues, and address other aspects of your physical health. This technique is used to treat sleeping disorders, lack of appetite, pain, and mood disorders. Because it relaxes you, shiatsu can also help reduce inflammation and stress-related health problems.

Structural Integration

Structural Integration, a form of bodywork, focuses specifically on the fascia, or connective tissues, that is inside your body. Fascia can be found surrounding all your nerves, organs, blood vessels, individual muscles, and groups of muscle. It binds these things together while still allowing movement.

While fascia should be elastic and move freely, it can become tight and dense over time, due to strain, injury, and repetitive motion. When it loses its elasticity, it pulls your frame out of alignment, causes pain and inflammation, and leads to fatigue.

By lengthening, stretching, and softening these tissues, Structural Integration seeks to restore movement, enhance blood flow, and improve your posture. This therapy can reduce pain, promote relaxation, and treat many inflammatory disorders.

Support Groups

Support groups are a form of talk therapy that involves groups of people coming together regularly to discuss shared experiences or get help with similar problems.

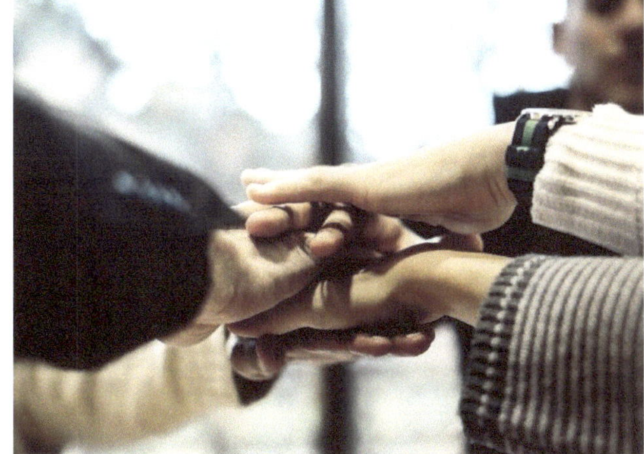

Participants receive advice, support, and encouragement, which can be helpful in addressing the psychological and emotional aspects of healing.

There are self-help groups for many different issues, including mental illness, chronic diseases, personal growth, and family support, as well as addiction counseling.

Support groups are beneficial for receiving acceptance, encouragement, and understanding about a particular problem. Sharing stories and expressing emotions can allow you to work through feelings from traumatic events.

By helping others in the group, you also gain a sense of pride and control. Participants often feel less stressed and more able to cope with their problems, which can lead to overall improved wellness.

Therapeutic Touch

Therapeutic touch combines techniques from several medical traditions to heal energy and enhance wellness. A practitioner passes his or her hands lightly over your body, not actually touching you, and detects any blockages in your energy pathways. The goal is to restore balance and energy to the energy surrounding the patient.

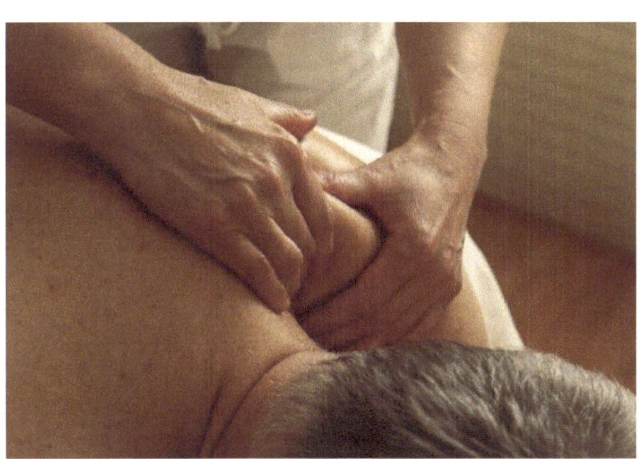

Therapeutic Touch creates a sense of relaxation, making it an effective treatment for many stress-related disorders. It can be used to reduce pain and stress as well as enhance mood, improve sleep and circulation, and reduce negative thoughts.

Traditional Chinese Medicine

Traditional Chinese Medicine (TCM) is a system of healing and wellness developed in China many centuries ago. The guiding principles of TCM include supporting good and getting rid of evil, which includes how you treat your health.

The goal of TCM is to promote health by strengthening your body's natural systems and defenses. Practitioners focus on how your body interacts with and is affected by the world in which we live, and it nurtures the mind, body, spirit connection.

As previously mentioned, chi (qi) is the life energy of the body, and TCM uses techniques to unlock and use that chi to achieve wellness. TCM has many techniques, including acupuncture, cupping, moxibustion, herbal medicine, and nutrition, to promote wellness and prevent disease.

Traditional Chinese Medicine focuses on balance and energy to create harmony and wellness both within and with others.

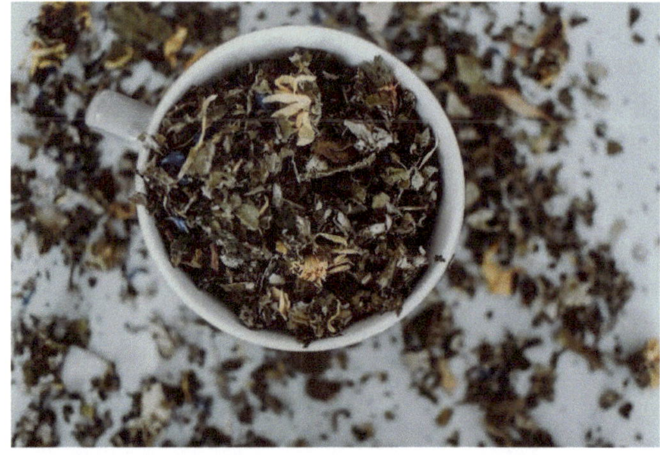

Traditional Japanese Medicine

Kampo is the name of Traditional Japanese medicine, which is essentially the study and practice of TCM in Japan. Since its introduction in Japan, though, TCM has been modified to include unique systems and techniques for diagnosis and treatment. Modern Kampo uses many of the traditional techniques of TCM but has a heavy emphasis on herbal medicines.

Traditional Korean Medicine

Korean medicine is that country's application and adaptation of TCM. In Korea, traditional medicine uses about 80 percent of the techniques used in China and Japan, but Korean medicine differs in a few ways.

The administration of herbal medicines and acupuncture treatments is different, with greater emphasis on individualization rather than standardization of treatment. Herbal treatments use less medicine than in TCM but more than is used in Japan.

Traditional Tibetan Medicine

Traditional Tibetan Medicine may be the foundation of all other eastern traditions and originated in the Himalayas. It has since migrated not only to the rest of China, Japan, and Korea but also to influence traditions in Russia, India, Europe, and North America.

Tibetan medicine predates Buddhism in that country, but over the centuries, it has evolved to include aspects of TCM, Ayurveda, and Persian medicine.

Tibetan medicine focuses more on the universal elements of space, air, fire, water, and earth than other Asian traditions. Illness is believed to be the result of mental poisons aversion, attachment, and ignorance. Most treatments involve diet and lifestyle changes, herbal medicines, and body manipulations.

Urine Therapy

Urine therapy, also known as autotherapy, utilizes your own urine to treat various illnesses. This therapy originated in India and has been used to treat many different conditions, including cancer.

Urine therapy involves either drinking one's own urine or applying it to the gums or skin. After you excrete it, urine is sterile and contains not only mostly water but also minerals, salts, enzymes, and hormones which can benefit your health.

Urine therapy is believed to boost immunity, prevent allergies, improve your heart health, prevent viral infections, and treat skin conditions such as acne. It has also been used to treat cold sores, arthritis, and even leprosy.

Visualization

Visualization, also known as guided imagery, uses your thoughts and imagination to relax and relieve symptoms. A trained practitioner teaches you how to relax and create vivid images in your mind that can help your body to heal itself.

The mental pictures created with visualization create a positive mindset about health, help you stay motivated to be healthy, and can help you identify your health goals and targets.

Visualization is an excellent tool for stress management, can help you sleep better and can help you cope with the pain and other symptoms of some chronic illnesses.

Zang-Fu Theory

Zang-fu theory is an aspect of TCM, which emphasizes a holistic understanding of how the body functions. Practitioners of zang-fu then apply techniques to treat the interactions between organs and how these influences your health.

Rather than identifying organs as the individual components of your body, this theory instead divides your entire body up into twelve organs, six zang, and six fu organs. When diagnosing problems, this theory looks for external signs to reveal what is happening internally, so that it can be addressed.

Because this theory was created before our anatomical understanding of the human body was fully known, the "organs" of zang-fu theory do not match what we think of today, but this way of thinking about the body yields a more holistic and integrated look at how our bodies perform and how various systems work together.

Final Thoughts

As you can now see, there is a wide range of alternative medicine techniques, traditions, and therapies that can be used in place of or to complement more conventional methods of healing. Alternative medicine is focused on prevention as well as seeking balance in one's life and health.

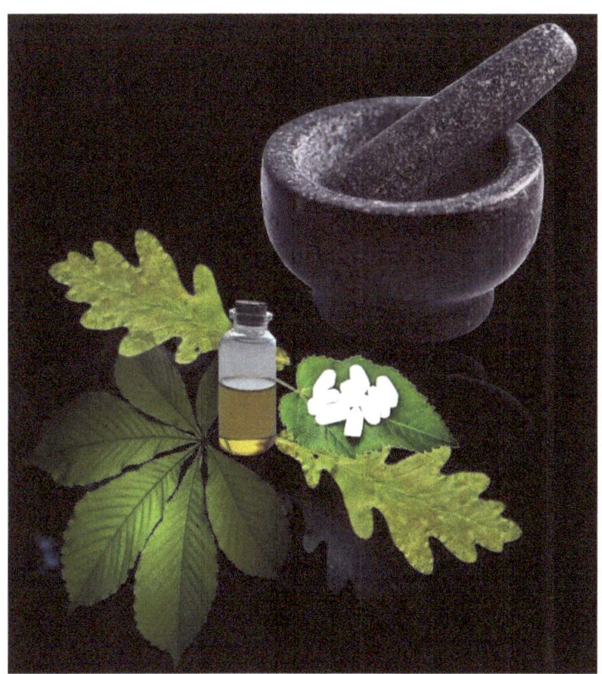

The techniques often promote your body's own ability to heal itself.

Alternative medicine therapies emphasize holistic approaches to wellness, recognizing that mental, physical, and emotional health all influence one another.

The philosophical and spiritual beliefs and principles that guide these healing methods can help you better understand their applications and their possible uses.

Choosing alternative medicine over conventional therapies, or complementing your conventional treatment with these techniques, gives you more options for your health and greater control how you achieve your personal well-being.

Always speak with your primary care doctor before using any alternative medicine options.

Stay well and take care!

About the Author

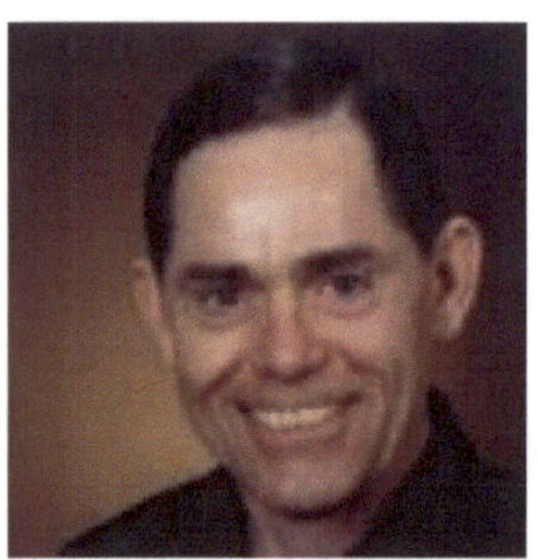

I have published numerous books on Amazon (both for Kindle and in paperback), along with other publishing platforms.

While most of my books are on health and fitness in general, I also write on baby boomer and older citizen health issues and have a recent interest in creating and printing journals/ planners and other printable products.

Besides my own writing, I also ghostwrite ebooks, books, reports, articles, blogs and do Kindle conversions for clients on a variety of topics.

Go to my website at http://ronknesswriting.com for more information or to submit a quote. For a complete list of my books, go to https://www.amazon.com/Ron-Kness/e/B0072M6PYO.

Today my wife and I are retired from our careers and live in San Tan Valley, AZ. I now write as a retirement business where you'll find me happily sitting in my office typing away on my laptop as I work on my next book or ghostwriting project . . . that is if we are not traveling on a cruise ship - our new-found mode of travel.